# FASTING GIRL

Simple guide on how women can lose weight,
balance hormones and become super strong

By

## Dr. Stacy Rose

**Remarks**


Simple, Concise for any woman out there.

Jennifer Stones, PhD


I like the way Stacy writes her stuffs like it's a lecture note.

Sandra cook, CEO, BLU


Without much debate, this is a good masterpiece for a new comer on fasting.

Natalie Freeman, Actress

# CONTENTS

# CHAPTER ONE: THE HISTORY OF FASTING

Fasting is when you don't eat or drink for a certain amount of time, usually for religious or health reasons. Fasting is often credited to ancient Greece, but it was practiced religiously by people of all religions and around the world at the time.

fasting, restraint from food or drink, or both for well-being, ceremonial, strict, or moral purposes. The abstention can be complete or partial, prolonged, brief, or sporadic. Fasting has been advanced and polished from olden times overall by doctors, by the pioneers and supporters of numerous religions, by socially assigned people (e.g., trackers or possibility for commencement customs), and by people or gatherings as a statement of dissent against what they accept are an infringement of social, moral, or political standards.

## Medical fasting

Fasting has been used as a treatment method since at least the fifth century BCE when the Greek physician Hippocrates advised patients with certain illness symptoms to avoid eating or drinking. A few doctors perceived a fasting impulse, by which patients in specific illness states normally experience a deficiency of hunger. A few doctors accepted that controlling food during such states was pointless and potentially even negative since fasting was believed to be a significant regular piece of the recuperation interaction.

A comprehension of the physiological impacts of fasting started to develop in the last option part of the nineteenth 100 years when a portion of the main coordinated investigations of fasting was done in creatures and people. Fasting techniques became increasingly sophisticated and diverse in the 20th century as more information about nutrition and the body's nutritional requirements emerged. Fasting, for instance, was practiced in a variety of settings, including at home, in a hospital, in a clinic, and as a treatment and prevention method. Some methods of fasting, particularly those used to treat chronic diseases, lasted longer than a month, allowed only water or calorie-free tea to be consumed, and included exercise and enemas. Other methods, known as modified fasting, allowed for 200 to 500 kilocalories per day (adults need between 1,600 and 3,000 kilocalories per day, depending on age, gender, and level of activity) and sometimes included psychological or spiritual therapy; contingent upon the specific strategy utilized, calories as a rule were as bread, vegetable stock, natural product squeeze, honey, or milk. Changed fasting was recognized from an exceptionally low-calorie diet, which permitted as much as 800 kilocalories each day and regularly was pointed toward prompting significant weight reduction. A 24-hour fast followed by a 24-hour regular calorie intake was an example of intermittent fasting, which involved cyclic periods of calorie restriction.

By the 21st hundred years, even though fasting was relevant in certain occasions of sickness, like in specific intense illnesses (especially when joined by a deficiency of hunger), whether fasting in different examples was valuable to human well-being stayed muddled. For instance, whereas studies on humans showed that 15-day intermittent fasting improved insulin-mediated glucose uptake into tissues, studies on rodents showed that long-term fasting promoted glucose intolerance and the release of harmful oxidants from tissues.

**Fasting and religion**

In the religions of old people groups and civilizations, fasting was a training to get ready people, particularly clerics, and priestesses, to move toward the divinities. In the Hellenistic mystery religions, it was believed that the gods would only show their divine teachings in dreams and visions after a fast that needed complete devotion from devotees. Among the pre-Columbian people groups of Peru, fasting frequently was one of the necessities for repentance after an individual had admitted sins before a cleric. In many societies, the training was viewed as a way to mollify an irritated divinity or to help with reviving a god who was accepted to have died (e.g., a lord of vegetation).

A vision quest was preceded and followed by fasting in the religions of some Native American tribes. Among the Evenk of Siberia, shamans (strict personages remembered to have the ability to recuperate and to impart clairvoyantly) frequently accepted their underlying dreams not with a journey yet rather after an unexplained sickness. But they fasted and trained themselves to see more visions and control spirits after the first vision. In the past, major seasonal-related ceremonies were preceded by fasting during retreats by priestly societies of Pueblo Indians in the American Southwest.

Fasting for unique purposes or previously or during extraordinary holy times stays a quality of significant religions of the world. In Jainism, for instance, fasting as per certain endorsed runs and rehearsing specific sorts of contemplation prompts dazes that empower people to separate themselves from the world and arrive at an extraordinary state. Fasting is a part of the meditation practices of some Theravada Buddhist monks. For a variety of reasons, Hindu sadhus (holy men) in India are admired for their frequent personal fasts.

Among the Western religions, just Zoroastrianism forbids fasting, in light of its conviction that such a type of plainness won't help with fortifying the devotion in their battle against evil. Judaism, Christianity, and Islam, the other Western religions, emphasize fasting during specific times. Judaism, which developed numerous dietary regulations and practices, observes several annual fast days, primarily on days of penitence (like Yom Kippur, also known as the Day of Atonement) or mourning. Christianity, particularly Eastern Orthodoxy and Roman Catholicism, has observed a 40-day fast during Lent, a spring penitential season preceding Easter, and Advent, a penitential season preceding Christmas. Since the Second Vatican Council (1962–65), the observance among Roman Catholics has been altered to allow for more individual choice, with obligatory fasting only occurring on Ash Wednesday and Good Friday during Lent. Protestant houses of worship for the most part pass on the choice too quick to individual church individuals. The long stretch of Ramadan in Islam is a time of contrition and complete fasting from daybreak to sunset.

# CHAPTER TWO:  BENEFITS OF FASTING FOR WOMEN

When attempting to lose weight, women over 50 may encounter difficulties. This can come from a few things. Frequently, a slowed metabolism is to blame. The slender muscle you have, the faster  your digestion becomes. However, as we get older, we often become less active and lose lean muscle mass. The outcome? Difficult muscle versus fat that simply will not appear to move.

Since the beginning of the year, Elizabeth has been going without food. Five months into the discontinuous fasting venture she posted, "The young lady on the left was continuously grinning, however, was never really content with herself, while the young lady on the right has a newly discovered love and appreciation forever, so her grin radiates certified bliss.

What five months of consistent fasting has accomplished for me still amazes me. For what it's worth with all the other things throughout everyday life, there are continuously going to be obstacles en route, however, it's what you decide to do after that obstacle that will have the effect between arriving at your objective or staying stale.

I'm so glad I found this way of life, and I'm grateful to you guys for inspiring me to keep going day after day.

For women, fasting can have a significant positive impact on numerous aspects of their health. The following are some major advantages:

1. Weight reduction: Women who want to lose weight can benefit from fasting. By limiting calorie consumption during fasting periods, the body takes advantage of putting away fat for energy, prompting weight reduction.

2. Hormonal Equilibrium: Fasting can assist with adjusting chemical levels in ladies. It can control insulin awareness and work on the body's reaction to insulin, which is significant for chemical guidelines, particularly in conditions like polycystic ovary disorder (PCOS).

3. Increased Sensitivity to Insulin: Women's insulin sensitivity can be improved through fasting, lowering their risk of insulin resistance and type 2 diabetes. Stabilizing blood sugar levels and improving metabolic health as a whole may result from this.

4. Upgraded Autophagy: Fasting triggers a phone cycle called autophagy, where the body purges and reuses harmed cells and cell parts. The risk of age-related diseases and healthy aging can both be aided by this process.

5. Expanded Energy and Mental Clearness: Women who fast may experience an increase in energy and mental clarity. It provides a steady and long-lasting fuel

source, easing the body's transition to using stored fat for energy.

6. Healthier Digestive System: Fasting offers the stomach-related framework a reprieve, permitting it to recuperate and fix. It can lighten stomach-related issues, for example, swelling, gas, and acid reflux.

7. Enhanced Immune Performance: The body's immune system relies heavily on the production of new white blood cells, which are sparked by fasting. In women, it may improve overall immune function and strengthen the immune system.

8. Decreased Aggravation: Fasting has been displayed to decrease irritation in the body. Persistent aggravation is related to different illnesses, and by diminishing it, fasting might work on ladies' general well-being and prosperity.

9. Physical, mental, and emotional health: Fasting has been shown to boost resilience, lower stress levels, and improve mood. Through practices of fasting, women may experience improved mental and emotional well-being.

10. Life span and Maturing: Fasting may have anti-aging effects and extend lifespans, according to some research. By advancing cell fixes and decreasing oxidative pressure, fasting might add to solid maturing in ladies.

It is essential to note that women with underlying health conditions or specific nutritional requirements should approach fasting cautiously and in consultation with medical professionals.

# CHAPTER THREE: MYTHS ABOUT FASTING

Fasting is associated with numerous myths. These fantasies have been rehashed frequently to the point that they are many times seen as dependable bits of insight. These myths include the following:

- When you fast, you go into a state known as "starvation."
- When you eat again, you will overeat.
- When you fast again, you will lose muscle.

- When you fast, you deprive your body of essential minerals.
- When you fast, hypoglycemia occurs because the brain needs glucose to function.
- It's just "crazy."

None of us would be alive today if they were true. Think about the consequences of using muscle as a source of energy. There were numerous days when there was no food available during prolonged winters. After the principal episode, you would be seriously debilitated. You would become so weak after several episodes that you would be unable to hunt or gather food. People couldn't have ever made due as an animal category. The better inquiry would be the reason the human body would store energy as fat if it wanted to consume protein all things considered. Naturally, the answer is that, contrary to what we discussed in the previous post, it does not cause muscle loss. It was merely a legend. Another persistent myth asserts that glucose is necessary for brain cells to function properly. This is inaccurate. Human cerebrums, remarkable among creatures, can involve ketones as a significant fuel source during delayed starvation, permitting the protection of protein-like skeletal muscle. Again, think about what would happen if glucose was essential to survival. People wouldn't make due as an animal category. Following 24 hours, glucose becomes drained and we become rambling morons as our minds shut down. Our astuteness, our main benefit against wild creatures, starts to vanish. People would have before long become wiped out. Fat is essentially the body's approach to putting away food energy as long as possible, and glucose/glycogen is the momentary arrangement. At the point when transient stores are drained, the body goes to its drawn-out stores without issues.

Think about a similarity. A refrigerator is used for short-term storage, while a freezer is used for long-term storage. Assume that three times each day, regularly, we go to the market to purchase food. The remainder is stored in the freezer, while some are stored in the refrigerator. Before long one cooler isn't sufficient, so we purchase another, then, at that point, another. Over a time of many years, we have ten coolers, and no place else to put them. Food in the cooler doesn't get eaten because three times each day, we purchase more food. There is no great explanation to let the food out of the cooler. What would happen if we decided to stop buying food one day? Would staying hungry cause everything to shut down? Nothing could be further from reality. To begin, we would empty the refrigerator. Then the food, so painstakingly put away in the cooler would be delivered.


As a result, in the body, glucose is used for short-term energy, and fat is used to store energy for long periods (the freezer). When there is a lot of glucose available, fat is not burned. Over many years of bountiful glucose, fat stores multiply. What might occur assuming glucose was abruptly inaccessible? Would staying hungry cause everything to shut down? Nothing could be further from reality. Energy, so painstakingly put away as fat, would be delivered.

Starvation mode, as it is prevalently known, is the secretive boogieman consistently raised to drive us off from missing even a solitary feast. For more than one year, around 1000 dinners are consumed. This amounts to 60,000 meals served over 60 years. To feel that avoiding 3 dinners of the 60,000 will some way or another cause hopeless damage is just crazy. The breakdown of muscle tissue occurs at extremely low body fat levels, around 4%. The majority of people do not need to be concerned about this. As of now, there could be no further muscle versus fat to be prepared for energy and lean tissue is consumed. The body of the human being has evolved to withstand brief bouts of starvation. Muscle is functional tissue, and fat is energy stored in cells. First, fat is burned. This is likened to putting away a tremendous measure of kindling yet choosing to consume your couch all things considered. It's dumb. Why do we think the body is so stupid? The body keeps building muscle until the amount of fat in the body is so low that it has no choice.

Investigations of substitute day-to-day fasting, for instance, show that the worry over muscle misfortune is to a great extent lost. Over 70 days, alternating daily fasting resulted in a weight loss of 6% and a fat mass loss of 11.4%. Slender mass (counting muscle and bone) didn't change by any stretch of the imagination. Huge upgrades were found in LDL cholesterol and fatty substance levels. Development of chemical increments to keep up with bulk. Despite the same amount of calories consumed, studies of eating a single meal per day revealed significantly greater fat loss. Importantly, there was no sign of muscle loss.

Another persistent myth about "starvation mode" is that our bodies "shut down" and basal metabolism drastically decreases. This also is exceptionally disadvantageous to the endurance of the human species. We would have less energy to hunt or gather food if our metabolism decreased after just one day of fasting. We are less likely to get food when we have less energy. As a result, we continue to deteriorate day after day, making it even more difficult for us to obtain food. This is an endless loop that the human species could not have possibly made due. It's dumb. Why do we think the body is so stupid? There are no animal species, including humans, that have evolved to require three meals daily. In a previous post, we learned that while fasting, resting energy expenditure (REE) increases rather than decreases. Digestion fires up; it doesn't close down.

It's hazy to me where this legend began. Because a daily caloric restriction causes a slower metabolism, it was assumed that this would only get worse as food intake fell to zero. This is off-base. If you depend on nourishment for energy, diminishing food will prompt diminished energy consumption, which will be matched by diminished energy use. Nonetheless, as food consumption goes to nothing, the body switches energy inputs from food to put away food (fat). This essentially expands the accessibility of 'food' and this is matched by an expansion in energy consumption.

So what occurred in the Minnesota Starvation Analysis? These members were not fasting. They were following a diet with fewer calories. Fasting-induced hormonal changes were not permitted. Because of a delayed time of bringing down food consumption, the body makes the change by lower TEE.

Everything changes when food admission goes to nothing (fasting). The body clearly can't bring TEE down to anything. The body now shifts its focus to burning the fat it has stored. After all, that is precisely the purpose for which it was placed. Our muscle versus fat is utilized for food when no food is free. It's not there for visual appeal.

Nitty gritty physiologic estimations show that TEE is kept up with or in some cases even expanded throughout a fast. TEE did not significantly decrease during 22 days of alternate daily fasting. There was no 'starvation' mode. There was no reduction in metabolic rate. While carbohydrate oxidation decreased from 53%, fat oxidation increased by 58%. This indicates that the body has begun to switch from burning sugar to burning fat without losing any energy overall. TEE rises by 12% after fasting for four days. Norepinephrine levels (adrenalin) soar 117% to keep up with energy. As the body switched to burning fat, fatty acids increased by over 372 percent. Insulin estimations diminished by 17%. Despite a slight drop, blood glucose levels remained within the normal range.

A low-calorie diet prohibits all of the extremely beneficial fasting adaptations.

notice how quickly the smallest amount of glucose reverses fasting's hormonal changes. Just 7.5 grams of glucose (2 teaspoons of sugar or scarcely a taste of a soda) is sufficient to invert ketosis. Very quickly in the wake of consuming glucose, the ketones beta-hydroxybutyrate and acetoacetate drop to barely anything, as do unsaturated fats. Both insulin and glucose rise.

What's the significance here? The body quits consuming fat. It has now gotten back to consuming the sugar that you are eating.

There are recurrent concerns that fasting could lead to overeating. There is a slight increase in calorie intake at the next meal, according to studies. Following a one-day quick, normal caloric admission increments from 2436 to 2914. Be that as it may, over the whole 2-day time frame, there is as yet a net shortage of 1958 calories. The extra calories did not even come close to making up for the day's lack of calories. From personal experience in our clinic, it appears that longer periods of fasting are associated with decreased appetite.

Does fasting deny the assemblage of supplements? The vast majority have more than adequate amounts of supplements. That is the general purpose. To dispose of a portion of these supplements - otherwise called fat. You can always take a multivitamin if you're worried about minerals and micronutrients. Concerns about nutrient deficiency can also be alleviated by following a different plan, such as alternate daily fasting (ADF).

The science is clear. The fantasies encompassing fasting were just lies.

# Chapter Four; Intermittent, Extended, alternate-day fasting

An eating plan that alternates between regular eating and fasting is known as intermittent fasting. Research shows that irregular fasting is a method for dealing with your weight and forestall — or even converse — a few types of infection. Yet, how would you make it happen? Is it secure, too?

**What is intermittent fasting?**

Intermittent fasting is all about when you eat, whereas many diets focus on what to eat.

When you practice intermittent fasting, you only eat at set times. According to research, eating only one meal a few days a week or fasting for a certain number of hours each day may have health benefits.

Johns Hopkins neuroscientist Imprint Mattson has read up irregular fasting for quite a long time. He claims that our bodies have evolved to be able to go days or even weeks without eating. In ancient times, before people figured out how to cultivate, they were trackers and finders who developed to get by — and flourish — for extensive stretches without eating. They needed to: Hunting game and gathering nuts and berries required a lot of time and effort.

Specialists note that even quite a while back, keeping a solid load in the US was simpler. Television was turned off at 11 p.m., and there were no computers. individuals quit eating since they headed to sleep. Much of the food was smaller. More individuals worked and played outside and, by and large, got more activity.

With web, television and other amusement accessible day in and day out, numerous grown-ups and kids stay alert for longer hours to sit in front of the television, look at virtual entertainment, mess around and visit on the web. That can mean sitting and nibbling the entire day — and the greater part of the evening.

Additional calories and less movement can mean a higher gamble of heftiness, type 2 diabetes, coronary illness and different diseases. Intermittent fasting, as demonstrated by scientific studies, may assist in reversing these trends.

There are a few unique ways of doing discontinuous fasting, however they are undeniably founded on picking normal time spans to eat and quick. You could, for instance, try eating only once every eight hours and fasting the rest of the time. Or on the other hand you could decide to eat just a single feast a day two days every week. There are several ways to run an intermittent fasting.

According to Mattson, the body begins to burn fat and consume  its sugar stores after going without food for several hours. He postulates this as metabolic exchanging.

"Discontinuous fasting is the typical eating design for most Americans, who eat all through their waking hours," Mattson says. " On the off chance that somebody is eating three meals per day, in addition to snacks, and they're not working out, then, at that point, each time they eat, they're working  on those calories and not consuming their body fats."

Discontinuous fasting works by drawing out the period when your body has copied through the calories eaten during your last meal and starts consuming body fat.

**Intermittent Fasting Plans**

Before beginning intermittent fasting, it is essential to consult your physician. When you receive their approval, the genuine practice is basic. You can choose a daily approach, which limits daily eating to one meal every six to eight hours. You could, for instance, try the 16/8 fast: eating for 8 hours and not eating for 16 hours.

Even though some people find it easy to stick with this routine over time, a study that wasn't specifically designed to look at intermittent fasting found that restricting your eating time each day doesn't stop weight gain over time or help you lose a lot of weight. According to the findings of that study, eating fewer large meals or eating more smaller meals may be linked to a reduction in weight gain or even weight loss over time.

One more irregular fasting plan, known as the 5:2 methodology, includes eating consistently five days every week. For the other two days, you restrict yourself to one 500-600 calorie feast. A model would be if you decided to eat ordinarily on each day of the week aside from Mondays and Thursdays, which would be your one-feast days.

Fasting for longer periods, such as 24 hours, 36 hours, 48 hours, or 72 hours, is not always better for you and may even be harmful. Going excessively lengthy without eating could  urge your body to begin putting away more fat in light of starvation.

Mattson's exploration demonstrates the way that it can require two to about a month before the body becomes familiar with irregular fasting. You could feel eager or crotchety while you're becoming accustomed to the new daily schedule. Yet, he notices, research subjects who endure the change time frame will more often than not stay with the arrangement since they notice they feel improved.

**What can I eat while intermittent fasting?**

During the times when you're not eating, water and zero-calorie drinks, for example, dark espresso and tea are allowed.

According to research, if you fill your mealtimes with high-calorie junk food, supersized fried foods, and treats, you are unlikely to lose weight or become healthier.

Yet, a few specialists like about discontinuous fasting that it takes into consideration a scope of various food sources to be eaten — and delighted in. Sharing great, nutritious food with others and enjoying the supper time experience adds fulfillment and supports great wellbeing.

Most sustenance specialists see the Mediterranean eating regimen as a decent plan of what to eat, regardless of whether you're attempting discontinuous fasting. You can barely turn out badly when you pick salad greens, solid fats, lean protein and mind boggling, crude sugars like entire grains.

## Intermittent Fasting Benefits

The intermittent fasting periods do more than just burn fat, according to research. "When changes occur with this fasting approach, it affects the body and brain," Mattson explains.

One of Mattson's examinations distributed in the New Britain Diary of Medication uncovered information about a scope of medical advantages related with the training. These incorporate a more extended life, a less fatty body and a more honed mind.

According to him, "intermittent fasting can protect organs against diseases like type 2 diabetes, heart disease, age-related neurodegenerative disorders, even IBS, and many cancers." "Many things happen during intermittent fasting."

Here are some intermittent fasting benefits research has revealed up until this point:

- Memory and the mind. Intermittent fasting has been shown to improve adult humans' verbal memory and working memory in animals.
- Heart Health. Irregular fasting further developed circulatory strain and resting pulses as well as other heart-related estimations.
- Physical performance. Young men who fasted for 16 hours lost fat while keeping their muscle mass. Mice that received food on alternate days demonstrated greater endurance when running.
- Obesity and diabetes type 2 In creature studies, discontinuous fasting forestalled weight. Furthermore, in six brief examinations, fat grown-up people shed pounds through irregular fasting. Beneficial effects may include: The majority of the research that has been conducted demonstrates that intermittent fasting can aid in weight loss by lowering fasting glucose, insulin, and leptin levels, as well as insulin resistance, leptin levels, and adiponectin levels. Certain examinations found that a few patients rehearsing discontinuous fasting with oversight by their primary care physicians had the option to invert their requirement for insulin treatment.
- Tissue Health. In creatures, discontinuous fasting diminished tissue harm in a medical procedure and further developed results.

**Is intermittent fasting safe?**

Certain individuals take a stab at intermittent fasting for weight the board, and others utilize the technique to address persistent circumstances like peevish entrail condition, elevated cholesterol or joint inflammation. Be that as it may, irregular fasting isn't ideal for everybody.

Williams focuses on that before you attempt discontinuous fasting (or any eating regimen), you ought to check in with your essential professional first. Certain individuals ought to avoid attempting irregular fasting:

- Teenagers and children under the age of 18
- Women who are either lactating or pregnant.
- Individuals with type 1 diabetes who take insulin. There have been no studies on people with type I diabetes, even though an increasing number of clinical trials have demonstrated that intermittent fasting is safe for people with type 2 diabetes. Mattson makes sense of, "Because those with type I diabetes take insulin, there is a worry that a discontinuous fasting eating example might bring about perilous degrees of hypoglycemia during the fasting time frame."
- Those with a background marked by eating problems

However, Williams asserts that those who can safely perform intermittent fasting and fall outside of these categories can adhere to the program indefinitely. She asserts, "it can be a lifestyle change that's benefiting."

Remember that discontinuous fasting might contrastingly affect various individuals. Converse with your PCP if you begin encountering strange tension, cerebral pains, queasiness or different side effects after you start irregular fasting.

## ALTERNATE-DAY FASTING

Alternate day fasting, or ADF for short, is a type of intermittent fasting in which people alternate between days when they fast and days when they don't. It typically follows a 24-hour cycle of periods of eating and periods of fasting.

Substitute day fasting (ADF) offers adaptability regarding planning fasting plans that suit individual inclinations and objectives. The following are a couple of well known substitute day fasting plans:

1. Fasting every alternate day: This plan includes shifting back and forth between fasting days and non-fasting days. On days when you fast, you either consume very few calories (less than 500) or none at all. On non-fasting days, you eat your ordinary feasts without explicit calorie limitations. Throughout the week, this pattern continues.

2. Alternate Day Fasting Modified: This approach takes into consideration some calorie consumption on fasting days, making it more reasonable for certain people. On days when you fast, you don't fast completely; instead, you eat 25 to 50 percent fewer calories than usual. On days when you are not fasting, you eat normally without counting calories.

3. Time-Confined Taking care of with Substitute Day Fasting: Time-limited feeding and alternate day fasting are included in this plan. It includes restricting the everyday eating window to a particular term (e.g., 8-10 hours) on both fasting and non-fasting days. This means that you eat everything you need to eat and burn calories within the allotted time, then you fast for the remaining hours.

4. 5:2 Fasting: In this variation of alternate day fasting, you eat normally five days a week and fast for two days that are not consecutive. While  fasting, you limit your calorie intake to 500-600 calories. You eat normally without any calorie restrictions on days when you are not fasting.

5. Alternate-day fasting: One meal a day (OMAD). The One Meal a Day approach and alternate day fasting are combined in this plan. On fasting days, you consume just a single dinner inside a short eating window (regularly 1-2 hours) and quick for the leftover hours of the day. You eat normally without any calorie restrictions on days when you are not fasting.

It is essential to keep in mind that fasting regimens ought to be tailored to meet the requirements, preferences, and health of each individual. It's fitting to talk with medical services experts or enlisted dietitians prior to beginning any fasting routine, particularly assuming you have hidden ailments or explicit nourishing prerequisites. In addition, for long-term success and adherence, it is essential to monitor your body's response and adjust the fasting plan as necessary.

## WHAT CAN I EAT WHILE OBSERVING ALTERNATE DAY FASTING PLAN

While noticing substitute day fasting, your food decisions on fasting days might change relying upon your particular fasting plan and objectives. The following are some general guidelines for what you can eat on days when you are fasting:

1. Extremely Low-Calorie Dinners: On days when you are not fasting, you can choose to eat very low-calorie meals if you want to consume some calories. Center around food sources that are supplement thick and low in calories. Leafy green vegetables, non-starchy vegetables, lean proteins like fish or chicken breast, and small amounts of healthy fats like olive oil or avocado are examples.

2. Protein-Rich Food varieties: Remembering protein for your fasting day dinners can assist you with feeling more full and keep up with bulk. Great wellsprings of protein incorporate eggs, tofu, lean meats, poultry, fish, and vegetables.

3. Foods High in Fiber: Eating fiber-rich food varieties can advance sensations of completion and backing stomach related wellbeing. Integrate wellsprings of fiber like entire grains, natural products, vegetables, and vegetables.

4. Hydration: Remaining all around hydrated is fundamental during fasting days. Drink a lot of water over the course of the day to keep up with hydration levels. Additionally, sweetener-free herbal teas and infusions can be consumed.

5. Beverages Low in Calorie: During periods of fasting, beverages with no calories, like plain black coffee and unsweetened herbal tea, are typically permitted. These can assist with checking hunger and give some assortment in taste without adding calories.

It's critical to take note of that the particular food varieties and calorie recompenses might change relying upon your fasting plan and individual necessities. On days of fasting, some people may choose to completely avoid food, while others may consume fewer calories. It's ideal to keep the rules set by your picked substitute day fasting plan or look for direction from a medical care proficient or enlisted dietitian to guarantee you are meeting your healthful requirements and remaining inside the boundaries of your fasting objectives.

## BENEFITS OF ALTERNATE DAY FASTING

Substitute day fasting (ADF) has been read up for its possible advantages. The following are a few potential advantages of intermittent fasting:

1. Weight reduction: Substitute day fasting can prompt calorie decrease and make a calorie shortage, which might add to weight reduction. It can help people accomplish and keep a better body weight by advancing fat misfortune while saving bulk.

2. Increased Sensitivity to Insulin: ADF has demonstrated promising effects on insulin sensitivity, which are beneficial to people with diabetes or insulin resistance. It might help keep blood sugar levels in check and make it easier for the body to use insulin.

3. Abatement of Inflammation: ADF might have calming impacts in the body. Persistent aggravation is connected to different ailments, and diminishing irritation can emphatically affect generally wellbeing and prosperity.

4. Improved Cell Fix and Autophagy: During fasting periods, the body can enter a condition of autophagy, which is a characteristic interaction where harmed cells

are stalled and reused. This cell fix instrument can assist with eliminating side-effects, work on cell capability, and possibly make hostile to maturing impacts.

5. Cardiovascular Wellbeing: ADF might emphatically affect cardiovascular wellbeing markers, including cholesterol levels, pulse, and fatty oil levels. It might assist with decreasing the gamble of coronary illness and work on generally cardiovascular wellbeing.

6. Potential advantages for the mind: A few examinations propose that discontinuous fasting, including ADF, may have mental advantages like superior concentration, mental lucidity, and neuroprotection. However, this area requires additional research.

7. Effortlessness and Adaptability: Because it involves alternating fasting and non-fasting days, ADF may be simpler than other methods of intermittent fasting. It gives adaptability in dinner arranging and can be adjusted to individual timetables and inclinations.

It is essential to keep in mind that every person's experiences and responses to alternate day fasting may differ. It might be more sustainable and beneficial to some people than to others. It's prescribed to talk with medical care experts or enlisted dietitians prior to beginning any fasting routine, particularly assuming you have basic ailments or explicit wholesome necessities.

In addition, alternate day fasting's long-term effects and potential dangers are still being investigated, necessitating additional research to fully comprehend its advantages and drawbacks.

## IS ALTERNATE DAY FASTING SAFE

Alternate-day fasting (ADF) can be ok for some people when done appropriately and under the direction of medical care experts. In any case, it may not be reasonable for everybody, and certain safeguards ought to be thought of. A few things to keep in mind are:

1. Individual Takeaways: ADF may not be reasonable for people with explicit ailments, like diabetes, dietary problems, or other constant medical issues. It's essential to talk with medical services experts, including specialists or enrolled dietitians, to decide whether ADF is proper for you.

2. Dietary Sufficiency: When adhering to ADF, it is essential to ensure that you meet your nutritional requirements on days when you are not fasting. Center around devouring a decent eating routine that incorporates different supplement thick food varieties. Assuming you can't meet your healthful requirements, dietary enhancements or customized feast plans might be suggested.

3. Hydration: Appropriate hydration is fundamental during fasting and non-fasting days. Make certain to hydrate over the course of the day to keep up with hydration levels. To avoid dehydration, this is especially important on days of fasting.

4. Monitoring: Focus on your body's signs and screen your prosperity all through the fasting system. ADF may not be right for you if you experience severe hunger, weakness, dizziness, or any other negative symptoms.

5. Personalization: ADF can be customized to fit individual necessities and inclinations. Changes in fasting term, recurrence, or calorie consumption on fasting days can be made to make it more reasonable and sensible for you.

6. Proficient Direction: Consult registered dietitians or healthcare professionals for advice that is tailored to your specific circumstances. They can assist with checking your advancement, guarantee security, and address any worries or questions you might have.

Keep in mind, the wellbeing and adequacy of any fasting routine rely upon different elements, including individual wellbeing, clinical history, and adherence to rules. It's vital to focus on your wellbeing and prosperity and go with informed choices in view of expert guidance.

# CHAPTER FIVE: GUIDELINES ON BREAKING A FAST

Care should be taken while breaking a quick so as not to overburden your stomach related framework. The best advantage of fasting is acknowledged when a quick is broken appropriately. Moving slowly  isn't simply kind to your body, however it permits YOU the chance to incorporate your freshly discovered clarity on your relationship to food.

During a quick, the body goes through a few organic changes. Proteins typically created by the stomach related framework have stopped being delivered or have been lessened extraordinarily, contingent upon the kind of quick performance, so presenting food gradually permits the body time to restore this compound creation.

The defensive bodily fluid coating of the stomach might be briefly lessened too, making the stomach walls more helpless against bothering until it additionally gets back to business as usual. This process is aided by a gradual reintroduction of foods, starting with those that are the simplest and easiest to digest. Substances known to be aggravating to the framework, for example, espresso and hot food varieties, should be stayed away from during the braking system.

Due to these organic changes, gorging promptly following a quick is a lot more regrettable than indulging at some other time. Your framework needs time to rearrange back to ordinary absorption and digestion. Not going to the appropriate lengths can bring about stomach squeezing, queasiness, and in any event, heaving. An illustration of this is given by a peruser of this site, Nita, who was able to share her experience of how not to break a quick.

The change time frame vital for breaking a quick depends on the length of the quick. Four days is thought of as satisfactory for any of the more drawn out diets, 1-3 days for more limited diets, and simply a day or so for one-day diets.

One more guideline is to require a portion of the quantity of days abstained to consider breaking. So a 4-day quick would require a multi day time span for the renewed introduction of food varieties.

**Foods to use for breaking a fast**

In the beginning, the most nutritious and simple foods are used to break a fast, adding more variety and complexity over time.

The kind of quick utilized will decide the sort of food varieties you use to break it. Juice and fruit are good for breaking a water fast, but they are not very good for breaking a juice or fruit fast.

Use the following list to help you decide when to introduce the various food groups. It starts with those that are simplest on the framework and can be presented from the get-go, and advances to those that ought to be added later.

Contingent upon the length of your quick, you might go through the rundown in one day or  4 days. Additionally, you are not required to consume everything on the list; it is merely a general guide.

- fruits and  juices
- vegetable
- yogurt (or other living, refined milk items), unsweetened

- lettuces and spinach (can involve plain yogurt as a dressing and top with new organic product)
- cooked vegetables and vegetable soups
- Cooked vegetables
- very much cooked grains and beans
- nuts and eggs
- milk items (non-refined)
- meats and whatever else

Any of the initial three things are  great for that underlying "breaking" of a fast, that first thing you eat; the easiest and most popular type is raw fruit.

Give close consideration to your body's responses to these "new" food sources. Keep an eye out for any negative reactions, which could indicate a mild allergy or that you've gone too far or too quickly. Feel for the impression of completion and quit eating by then. Start to prepare yourself to look for that sign, so you'll constantly know when your body is completely supported.

When breaking a fast, start with small meals every two or three hours and work your way up to larger meals with more time between them until you reach a "normal" eating pattern, like eating three meals and two snacks per day.

Chew food thoroughly. This is a good habit to form and will assist digestion greatly.

Try to get more good bacteria and live enzymes into your system. New, crude food sources are loaded with living catalysts great for your body and absorption. In addition to pills, naturally cultured and fermented foods like yogurt, sauerkraut, and miso contain probiotics, or "good" bacteria.

By and large, the accompanying four elements address what we are attempting to achieve while breaking a fast.

# CHAPTER SIX: GUIDES ON HOW TO START A FAST

While beginning a quick, it's vital to move toward it carefully and think about your singular requirements and conditions. Here are a few overall principles to assist you with beginning a quick:

1. Select a Fasting Mode: Choose the method of fasting that best suits your objectives and preferences. Normal choices incorporate irregular fasting (like 16/8 technique or substitute day fasting), expanded fasting (24 hours or longer), or time-limited taking care of. Research various techniques and pick the one that suits you best.

2. Clear Objectives: Characterize your objectives for fasting. Is it true or not that you are hoping to get in shape, work on metabolic wellbeing, or experience the possible advantages of fasting? Having clear objectives can assist you with remaining propelled and keep tabs on your development.

3. Make a plan: Before beginning a quick, plan your feasts and timetable in like manner. Choose the duration of your eating window and meal times if you are practicing time-restricted feeding. For longer diets, plan the term and consider any occasions or exercises that might be influenced by the quick.

4. Gradual Method: If you're new to fasting, starting slowly can be helpful. Begin by fasting for shorter periods, like 12 or 14 hours, and gradually lengthen them over time. This permits your body to change and assists you with measuring your capacity to bear fasting.

5. Hydration: Focus on hydration during your quick. To keep your body properly hydrated throughout the day, drink a lot of water. To help you stay hydrated, you can also drink herbal teas, black coffee, and electrolyte-rich drinks that don't have many calories or are high in them.

6. Adjusted Nourishment: While not fasting, center around consuming a reasonable eating regimen that gives satisfactory supplements. Incorporate various entire food sources, including organic products, vegetables, lean proteins, entire grains, and solid fats. This guarantees you're meeting your healthful necessities on non-fasting days.

7. Oversee Appetite and Desires: You may experience cravings and hunger during fasting. To control them, keep yourself occupied with activities, break your fast with mindful eating, and think about eating filling foods like protein, fiber, and healthy fats to keep you full.

8. Pay attention to Your Body: Adjust your approach to fasting based on what your body is telling you. Assuming you experience delayed distress, wooziness, shortcoming, or any extreme side effects, it could be important to break the quick and look for clinical counsel if necessary.

9. Responsibility and assistance: Consider joining on the web networks or finding fasting pals to share encounters, gain backing, and remain propelled. The

journey of fasting can be made more enjoyable and sustainable with the help of a support network.

10. Advice from a professional: Before beginning a fast, it's best to talk to doctors or registered dietitians if you have specific health concerns or medical conditions. They can give customized direction and guarantee fasting is ok for you.

Keep in mind, fasting isn't reasonable for everybody, and individual encounters might shift. When beginning a fast, it is essential to place your personal comfort, health, and well-being first.

# CHAPTER SEVEN: HEALTHY NUTRIENTS FOR WOMEN

Ladies have special healthful requirements. You can control cravings, manage your weight, have more energy, and look and feel your best by eating well throughout your life.

It can be challenging for any woman to keep a healthy diet because of the demands of family, work, or school, and the media's pressure to look and eat a certain way. Be that as it may, the right food can not just work on your temperament, support your energy, and assist you with keeping a sound weight, it can likewise uphold you through the various stages in a woman's life.

Many of us, especially women, frequently neglect our dietary requirements. You might feel that you're excessively occupied to eat well or used to putting the requirements of your family before your own. Or on the other hand maybe you're attempting to adhere to an outrageous eating routine that leaves you short on indispensable supplements and feeling testy, hungry, and coming up short on energy.

Ladies' particular necessities are in many cases dismissed by dietary exploration, as well. Nutritional studies typically use male subjects, whose hormone levels are more stable and predictable. As a result, the results may not always be relevant to women's needs or even be misleading. This can amount to serious deficiencies in your day to day nourishment.

While what turns out best for one lady may not generally be the most ideal decision for another, the significant thing is to assemble your eating regimen around your indispensable healthful requirements. These nutrition tips can assist you in remaining healthy, active, and vibrant throughout your ever-changing life, whether you want to combat stress or PMS, boost fertility, enjoy a healthy pregnancy, or ease the symptoms of menopause.

Certainly! Here are a few significant supplements that are especially helpful for ladies' wellbeing:

1. Iron: Iron helps prevent iron-deficiency anemia, so women need to get enough of it, especially during menstruation. Great wellsprings of iron incorporate lean meats, poultry, fish, vegetables, sustained grains, spinach, and tofu. Vitamin C-rich foods and iron-rich foods can both increase iron absorption.

2. Calcium: Calcium is important for keeping teeth and bones strong, as well as for how muscles work and how nerves communicate. Dairy items, braced plant-based

milk choices, verdant green vegetables (like kale and broccoli), and calcium-strengthened food varieties are superb wellsprings of calcium.

3. Folate (Folic Corrosive): Folate is significant for ladies of childbearing age, as it forestalls brain tube absconds during early pregnancy. It additionally upholds red platelet creation. Leafy green vegetables, legumes, fortified grains, citrus fruits, and folic acid supplements are all good sources of folate (especially for pregnant women).

4. Fatty Acids Omega-3: Omega-3 unsaturated fats, especially EPA (eicosapentaenoic corrosive) and DHA (docosahexaenoic corrosive), are helpful for heart wellbeing and cerebrum capability. Omega-3s are abundant in walnuts, flaxseeds, chia seeds, and fatty fish like salmon, mackerel, and sardines.

5. Vitamin D: Vitamin D is fundamental for calcium retention, bone wellbeing, and safe capability. The body makes vitamin D when it is exposed to sunlight. Fatty fish, fortified dairy products, and some mushrooms are food sources. Enhancements might be vital on the off chance that you have restricted sun openness.

6. Magnesium: Magnesium supports bone health, muscle function, and energy production in the body and is involved in hundreds of enzymatic reactions. Nuts, seeds, whole grains, legumes, leafy green vegetables, and dark chocolate are all good sources of magnesium.

7. Vitamin B12: Red blood cell production, nerve function, and DNA synthesis all depend on vitamin B12. It is mostly found in dairy, meat, poultry, fish, and other animal products. Vegetarians or people with restricted creature item admission might have to enhance with vitamin B12.

Keep in mind, it's vital to keep a reasonable and changed diet to guarantee you're getting every one of the fundamental supplements your body needs. If you have explicit wholesome worries or dietary limitations, it's prudent to talk with a medical services proficient or enrolled dietitian for customized direction.

# CHAPTER EIGHT: IMPLEMENTING FAT LOSS THROUGH FASTING

Fasting for fat loss can be a way to help you reach your weight loss goals. When using fasting to lose weight, follow these guidelines:

1. Pick a Fasting Strategy: There are different fasting techniques you can consider, for example, discontinuous fasting, substitute day fasting, or broadened fasting. Choose the method of fasting that best suits your preferences and way of life.

2. Calorie Shortfall: To lose fat, you want to make a calorie shortfall, and that implies consuming fewer calories than your body needs. Focus on eating whole, nutrient-dense foods during your eating windows or non-fasting days while being mindful of portion sizes and overall calorie intake.

3. Adjusted Nourishment: On days when you are not fasting, it is essential to give priority to eating a well-balanced diet. Incorporate different natural products, vegetables, lean proteins, entire grains, and

solid fats in your dinners to meet your supplement needs and back general well-being.

4. Pay attention to portions: While breaking your quick, focus on segment sizes to forestall indulging. Begin with more modest partitions and pay attention to your body's appetite and completion prompts.

5. Hydration: Keep a steady supply of water throughout the fasting period. Drink a lot of water during fasting and non-fasting periods to help with hydration and general prosperity.

6. Exercise: Integrate ordinary actual work into your daily schedule. Exercise can assist with consuming extra calories, support muscle development, and further develop good body posture. Find exercises you appreciate and take a stab at a mix of cardiovascular activity and strength preparation.

7. Screen Progress: Monitor your advancement by recording your weight, estimations, and body piece changes. You might be able to stay motivated and change your approach as a result of this.

8. Stability and consistency: Consistency is key while carrying out fasting for fat misfortune. Be consistent with your method of fasting and be patient with the process. Finding a strategy that you can stick with and enjoy over time is essential.

9. Proficient Direction: Assuming that you have any fundamental ailments or concerns, or on the other hand on the off chance that you're uncertain about how to carry out fasting securely and really, it's prescribed to talk with medical services experts or enrolled dietitians. They can give customized directions because of your singular necessities.

Keep in mind that while fasting can help you lose weight, your overall health and well-being should come first. Fasting may not be right for everyone, so listen to your body and make any necessary adjustments.

# CHAPTER NINE: HOW DO FASTING AND ENERGY LEVELS RELATE

Fasting for fat loss can be a way to help you reach your weight loss goals. When using fasting to lose weight, follow these guidelines:

1. Pick a Fasting Strategy: There are different fasting techniques you can consider, for example, discontinuous fasting, substitute day fasting, or broadened fasting. Choose the method of fasting that best suits your preferences and way of life.

2. Calorie Shortfall: To lose fat, you want to make a calorie shortfall, and that implies consuming fewer calories than your body needs. Focus on eating whole, nutrient-dense foods during your eating windows or non-fasting days while being mindful of portion sizes and overall calorie intake.

3. Adjusted Nourishment: On days when you are not fasting, it is essential to give priority to eating a well-balanced diet. Incorporate different natural products, vegetables, lean proteins, entire grains, and

solid fats in your dinners to meet your supplement needs and improve general health

4. Pay attention to portions: While breaking your quick, focus on segment sizes to forestall indulging. Begin with more modest partitions and pay attention to your body's appetite and completion prompts.

5. Hydration: Keep a steady supply of water throughout the fasting period. Drink a lot of water during fasting and non-fasting periods to help with hydration and general prosperity.

6. Exercise: Integrate ordinary actual work into your daily schedule. Exercise can assist with consuming extra calories, support muscle development, and further develop a good body posture.  Find exercises you appreciate and take a stab at a mix of cardiovascular activity and strength preparation.

7. Screen Progress: Monitor your advancement by recording your weight, estimations, and body piece changes. You might be able to stay motivated and change your approach as a result of this.

8. Stability and consistency: Consistency is key while carrying out fasting for fat misfortune. Be consistent with your method of fasting and be patient with the process. Finding a strategy that you can stick with and enjoy over time is essential.

9. Proficient Direction: Assuming that you have any fundamental ailments or concerns, or on the other hand on the off chance that you're uncertain about how to carry out fasting securely and really, it's prescribed to talk with medical services experts or enrolled dietitians. They can give customized detection directions because of your singular necessities.

Keep in mind that while fasting can help you lose weight, your overall health and well-being should come first. Fasting may not be right for everyone, so listen to your body and make any necessary adjustments.

# CHAPTER TEN: HOW WOMEN CAN GAIN ENERGY AND BALANCE HORMONES

Ladies can find multiple ways to acquire energy and equilibrium chemicals. Some options to think about are:

1. Adjusted Diet: Center around devouring a reasonable eating regimen that incorporates various supplements and food varieties. Integrate lean proteins, entire grains, natural products, vegetables, sound fats, and vegetables. Guarantee you're getting sufficient nutrients and minerals, including iron, calcium, magnesium, and B nutrients.

2. Glucose Guideline: Settle glucose levels by eating standard, adjusted dinners and snacks over the day. Incorporate a blend of complicated sugars, protein, and solid fats in your feasts to advance supported energy levels.

3. Hydration: Remain all around hydrated by drinking sufficient water over the day. Drying out can add to weariness and chemical awkward nature.

4. Oversee Pressure: Persistent pressure can upset the chemical equilibrium and lead to exhaustion. Practice pressure the executives' methods like profound breathing activities, contemplation, yoga, or taking part in exercises you appreciate. Create time for yourself and prioritize self-care.

5. Ordinary Activity: Regular exercise can help maintain hormone balance and give you more energy. Consolidate a blend of cardiovascular activity, strength preparation, and exercises that advance adaptability and stress decrease.

6. Sleeping well: Hold back nothing sufficient rest to help with chemical guidelines and energy levels. Practice good sleep hygiene, create a sleep-friendly environment, and establish a regular sleep schedule.

7. Foods that Balance Hormones: Hormone balance can be supported by certain foods. Include cruciferous vegetables like broccoli, cauliflower, and kale, foods high in antioxidants like berries, and dark chocolate, and foods high in omega-3 fatty acids like chia seeds, flaxseeds, and fatty fish in your diet.

8. Limit Alcohol and caffeine: Drinking too much alcohol and caffeine can make it hard to sleep, upset the balance of hormones, and make you feel tired. Limit your admission and be aware of their consequences for your energy levels.

9. Think about Enhancements: Ask your doctor or a registered dietitian about supplements that might help you keep your hormones in balance and have enough energy. This could include supplements made from herbs, minerals, or vitamins that are made just for you.

10. Look for Proficient Direction: Consider consulting with women's health specialists in the healthcare industry if you are experiencing significant hormonal imbalances or persistent fatigue. They can lead fitting assessments, present customized suggestions, and investigate expected fundamental causes.

Keep in mind, each lady's process is remarkable, and it's essential to pay attention to your body and make changes because of your singular necessities. To achieve optimal levels of energy and hormone balance, working with healthcare professionals can provide individualized guidance and support.